Introduction

The Story of the Cheeky tooth came about when Ella (6) had a tooth that just refused to come out. She called this tooth her Cheeky tooth and came up with the story.

With help from daddy and Granda Jim drawing some pictures the story of the Cheeky tooth was born

The Cheeky Tooth

By :- Ella Glennie

Illustrated by Jim "Granda Jim" Glennie

Published by Andrew Glennie
ISBN 978-1-4717-1237-1

This is Ella

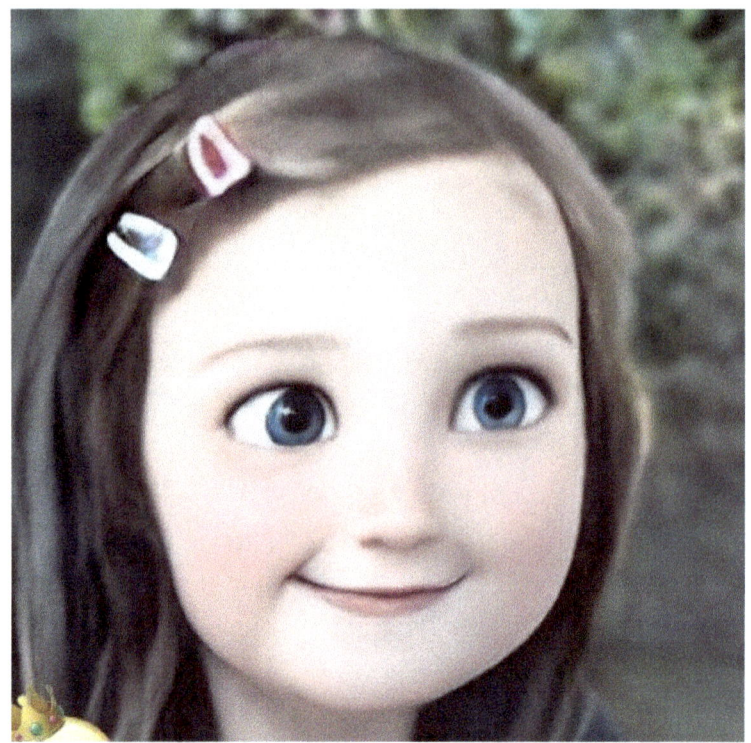

Ella is 6 years old. Ella brushes her teeth every morning after she has breakfast and again every night before she goes to bed.

Ella really looks after her teeth

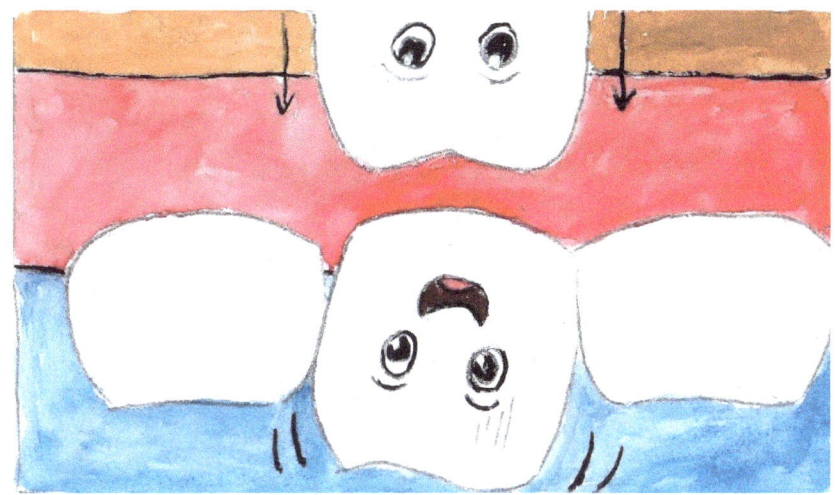

Ella has a Wobbly tooth. It is time for her baby tooth to fall out and be collected by the tooth fairy so Ella's grown up tooth can come through.

Ella wobbled and wobbled it, but it wouldn't fall out

Ella's tooth was The Cheeky Tooth

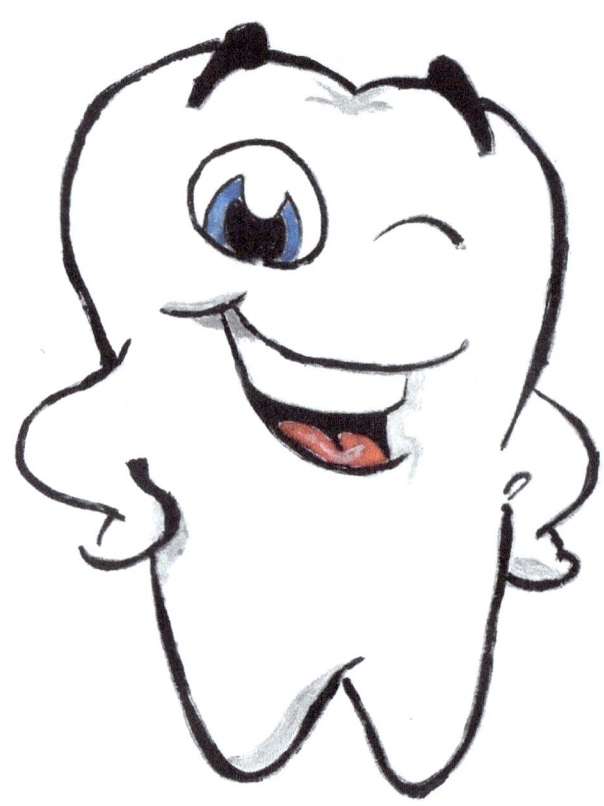

Ella ate some corn on the cob. The Cheeky Tooth said "NOPE I'm not coming out, I like it in here"

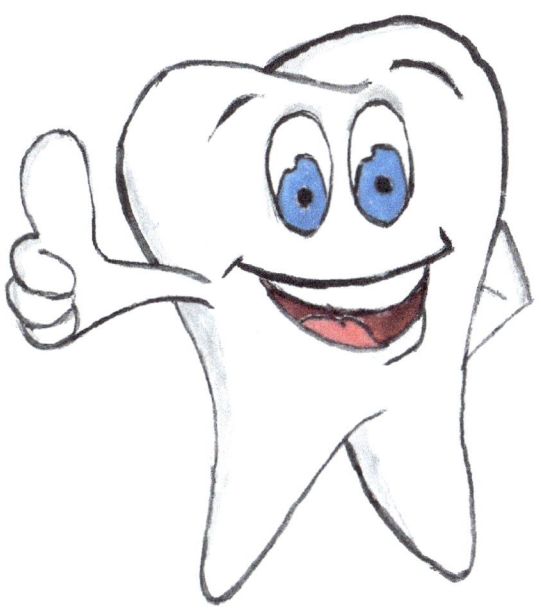

The Tooth

Fairy came by that night looking for the tooth, but she had to leave without The Cheeky Tooth as it didn't fall out.

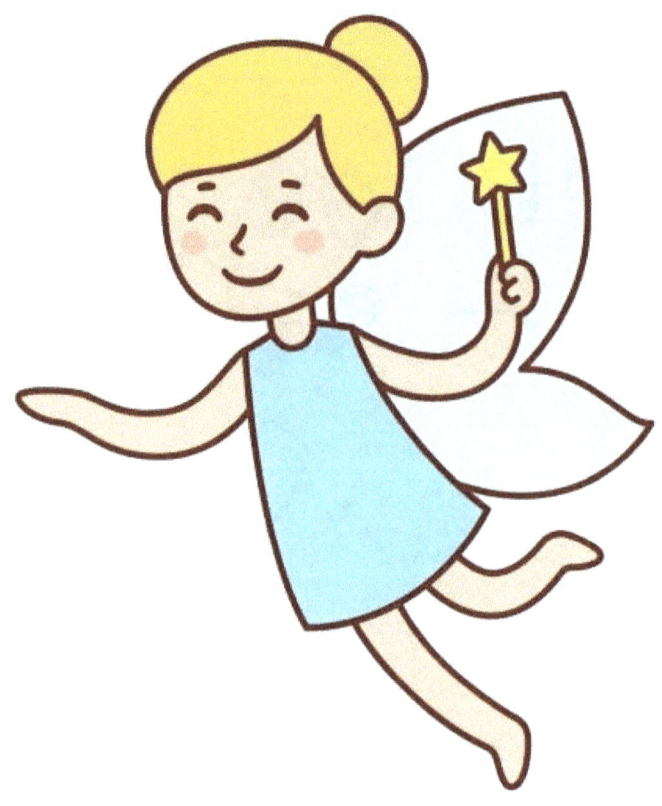

The next day Ella ate an apple, but The Cheeky Tooth said "I'm happy in here I'm not coming out"

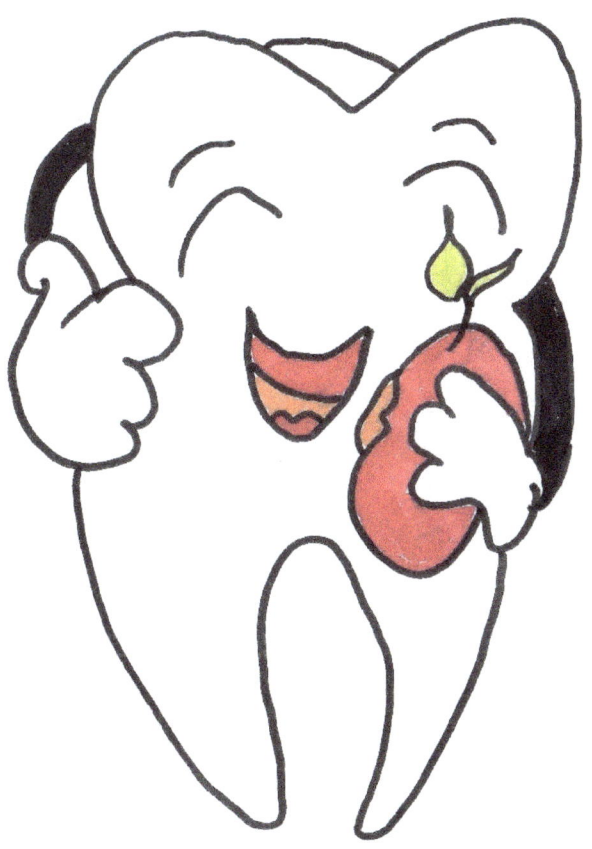

Fairy came again that night,

The Tooth

but The cheeky Tooth wasn't under Ella's pillow, so off she flew again empty handed

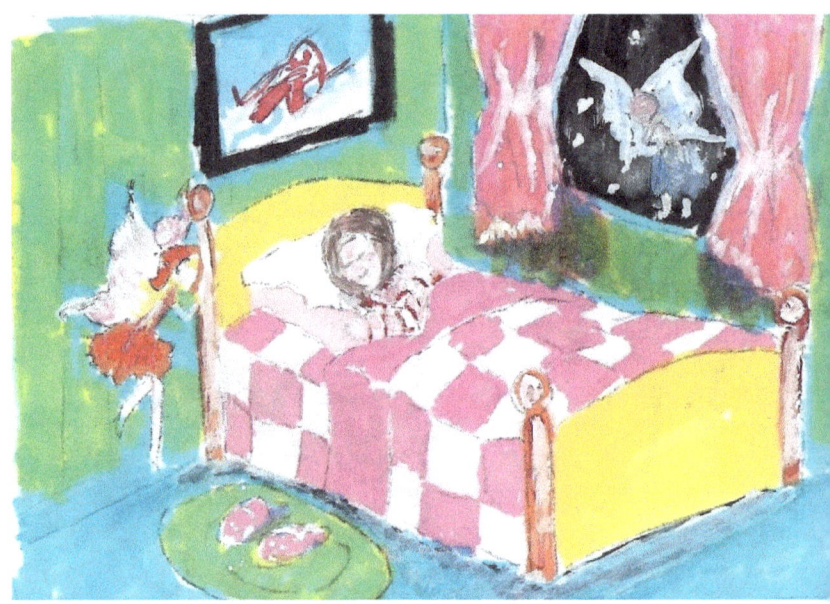

The next day Ella ate a ham sandwich and The Cheeky Tooth said "Yum Yum, this is

tasty but I'm still not leaving" while he danced and spun around

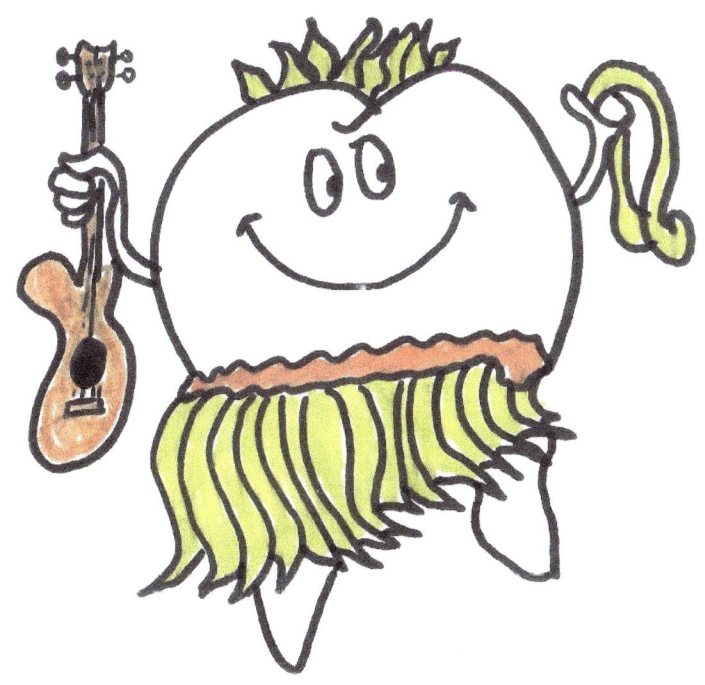

Fairy came round again that night, hoping to get the tooth this time, she flew into Ella's bedroom.

The Tooth

Ella was fast asleep so The Tooth Fairy looked everywhere

Still no cheeky tooth to be found.

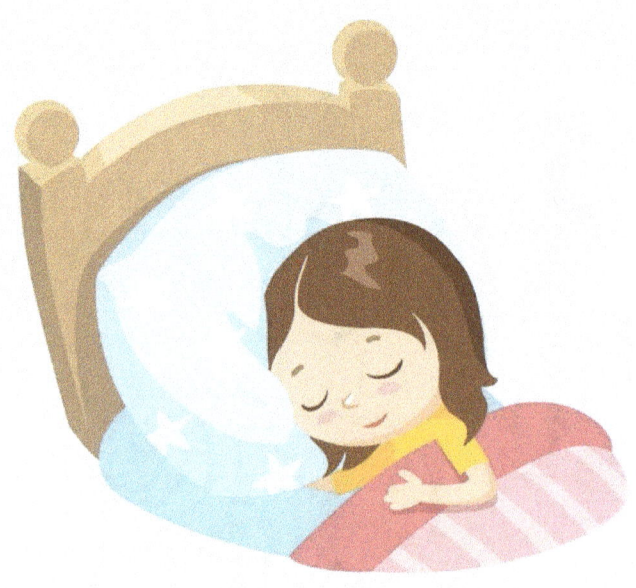

But then The Cheeky Tooth peeked out and said.

"I'm still not coming with you I like it here"

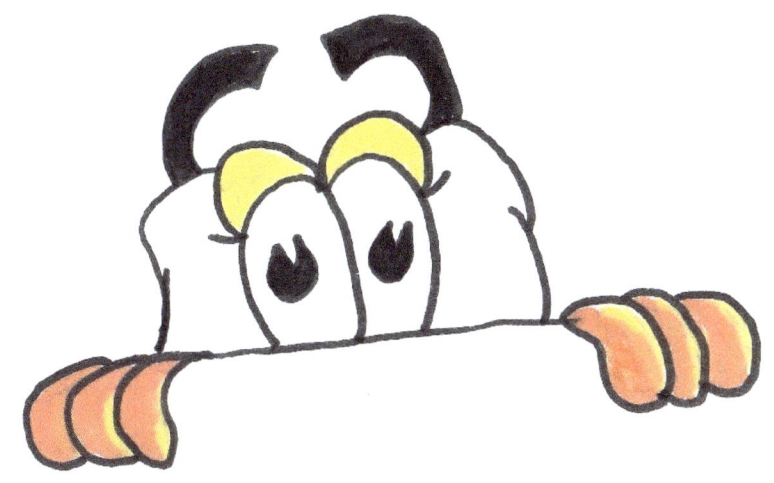

Fairy was getting cross now,
She was so cross her hair changed colour,
Is it any wonder she was cross, have you

The Tooth

seen how much it costs to fly these days
fuel prices are through the roof.

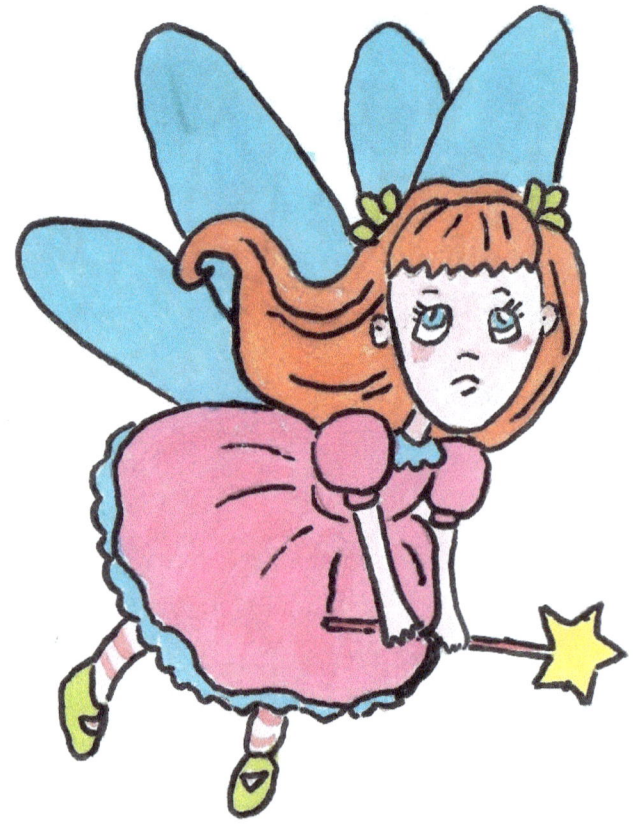

Ella was becoming used to having a
cheeky tooth now though and made up a
poem.

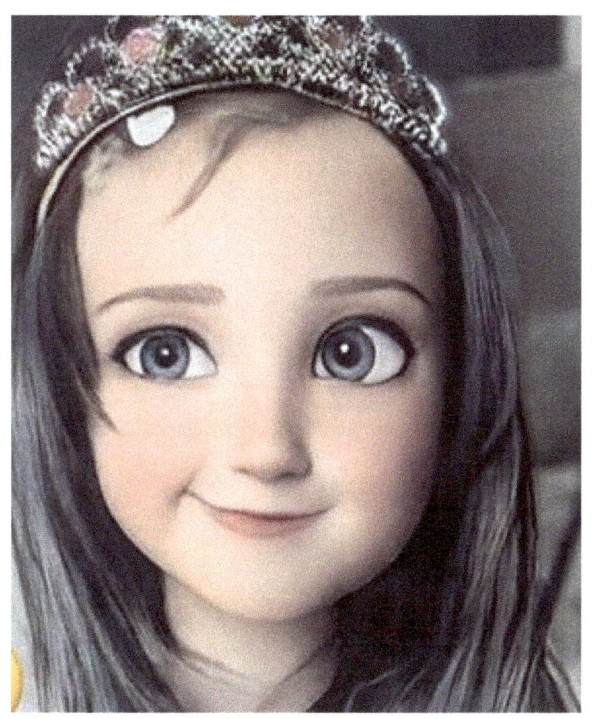

"I have a cheeky tooth at the top of my mouth

I wobble it and wobble it, but it won't fall out.

Ella ate a banana and still the cheeky tooth held on tight.

he sang "I am a cheeky tooth, I'll wibble and I'll wobble but I won't fall out"

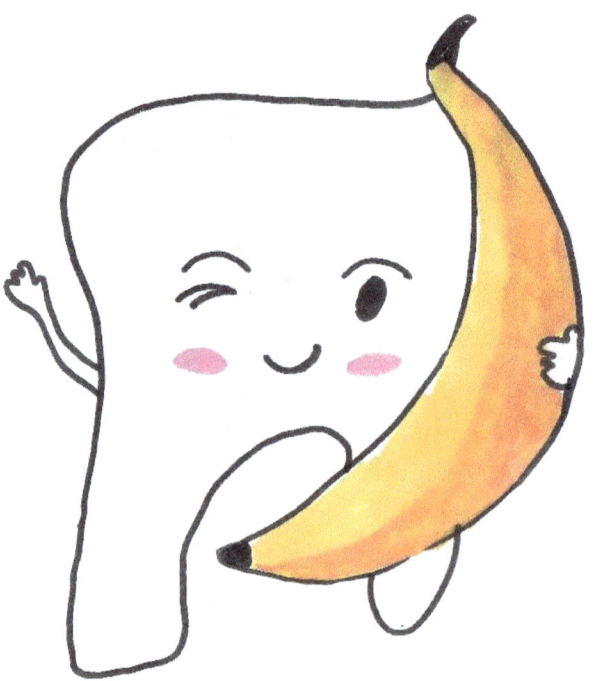

The Tooth Fairy didn't come by that night, with all the flying backward and forward

she was worn out, so instead she sent the
work experience guy

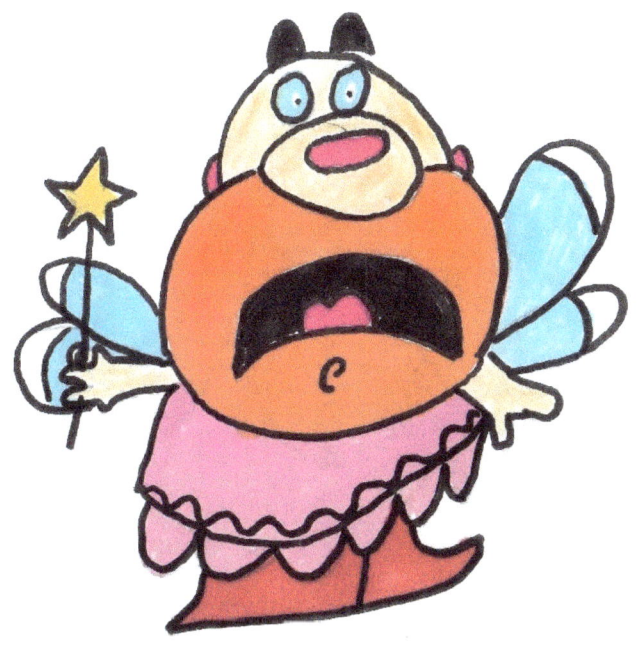

But the cheeky tooth just waved and
chanted. "I'm staying in here, I'm staying in
here".

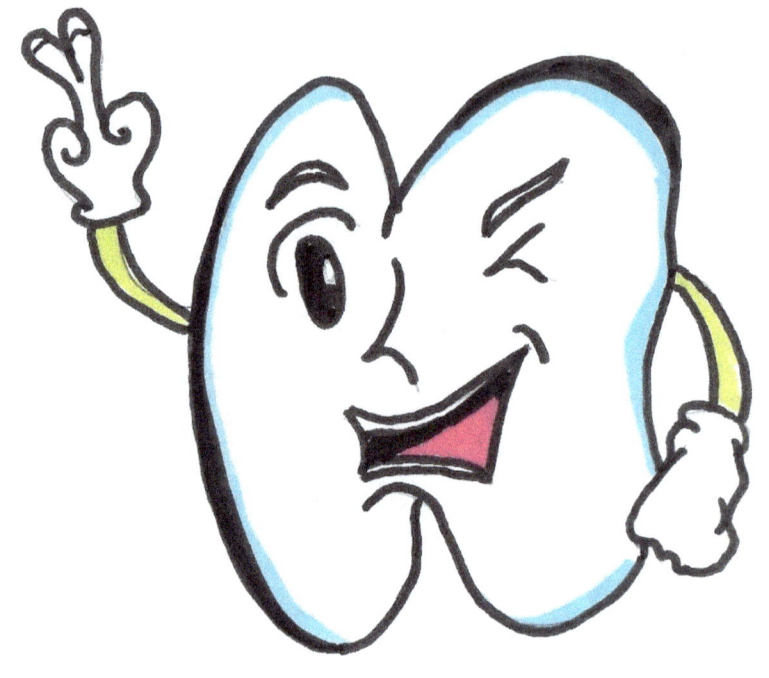

The very next day Ella had toast for breakfast, The Cheeky Tooth started singing.

"I am a cheeky tooth, I love being fed, I won't fall out before Ella goes to bed"

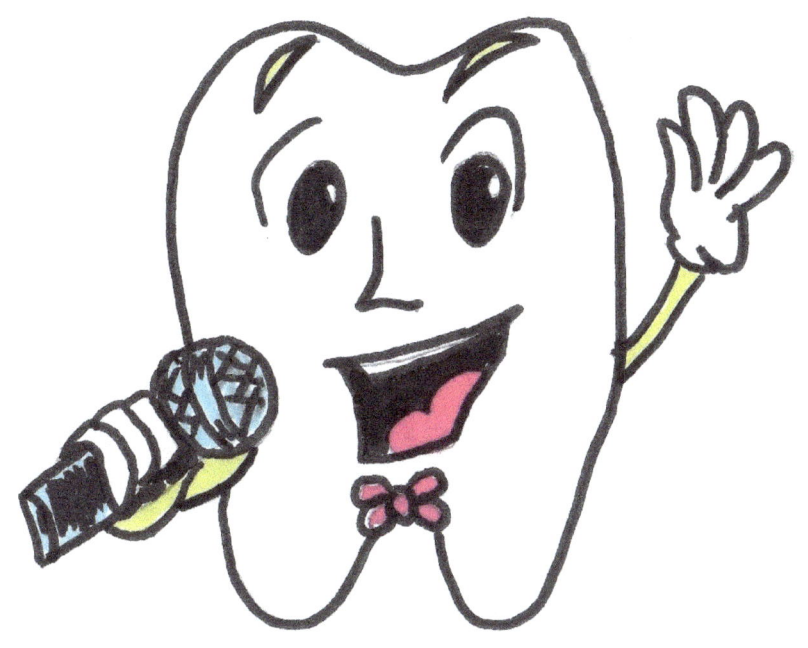

When breakfast was finished Ella went to brush her teeth as usual.

The Cheeky Tooth wasn't paying attention with all his singing though and forgot to hang on and out he fell when the toothbrush buzzed by.

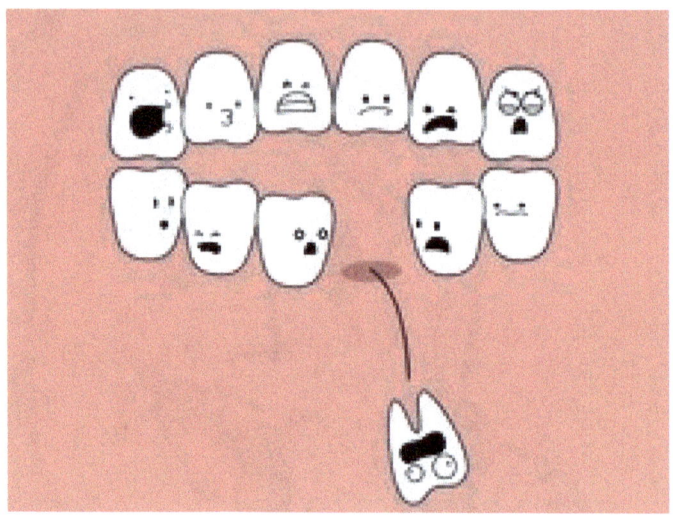

Ella took The Cheeky Tooth and wrapped him up warm and cosy and left him under her pillow and went off to school

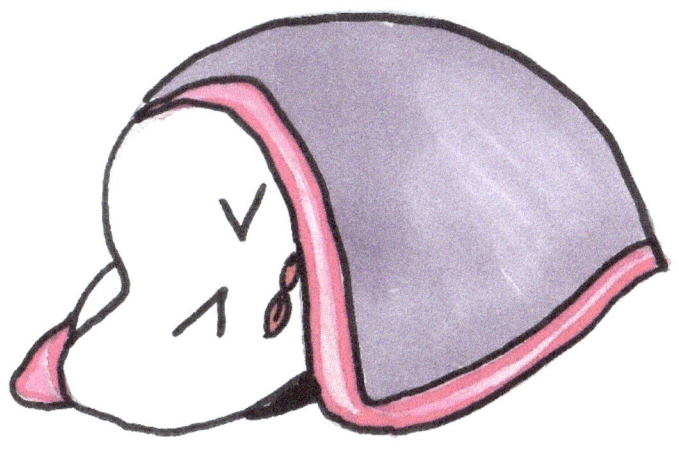

That night Ella checked he was there safe
and sound and went off to sleep. Just after
midnight The Tooth Fairy stopped by,

hoping to find The Cheeky Tooth, and this time she did.

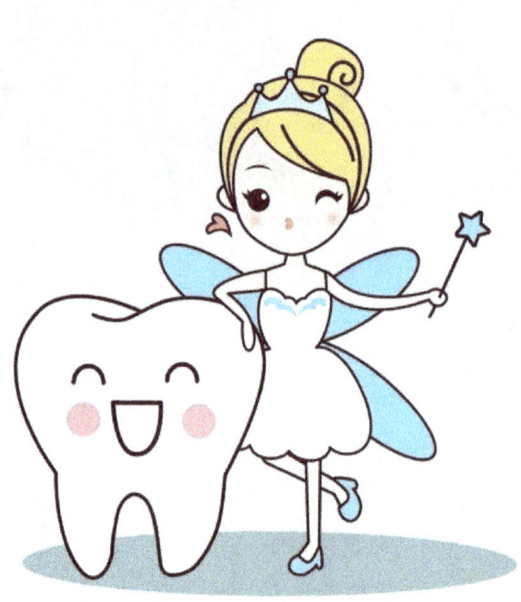

The Tooth Fairy was really happy to finally find the tooth and left Ella a shiny gold

coin, and Ella was happy that her tooth
finally fell out.

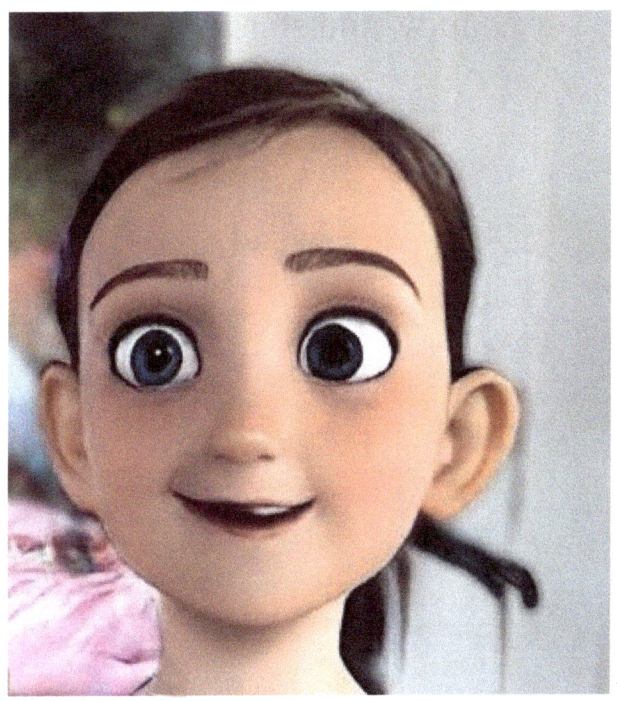

The Cheeky Tooth was a bit afraid of where
he was going to go now, but when he got

to The Tooth Fairy's castle and found he
had lots of other baby teeth to play with
he was very happy, and still very cheeky

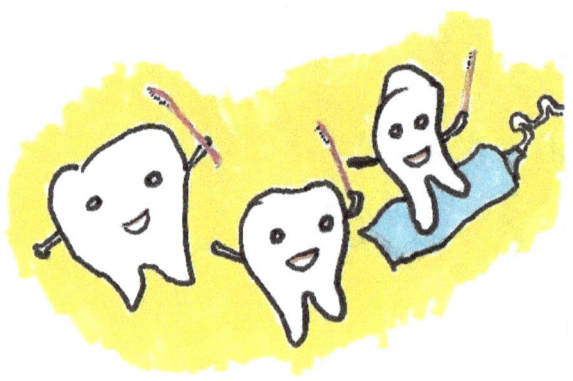

Thank you all for reading the Cheeky Tooth.

And thank you to Granda Jim for the drawings

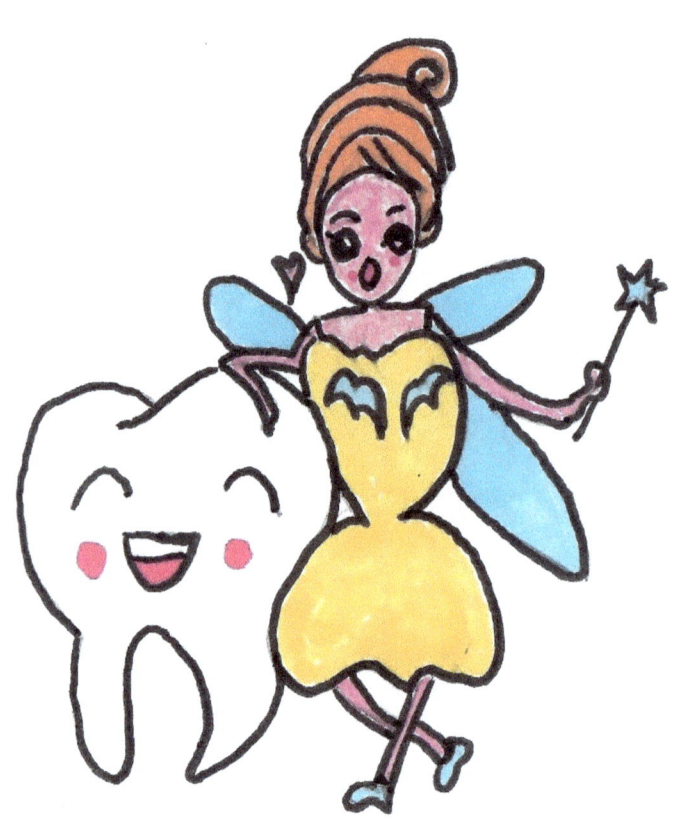

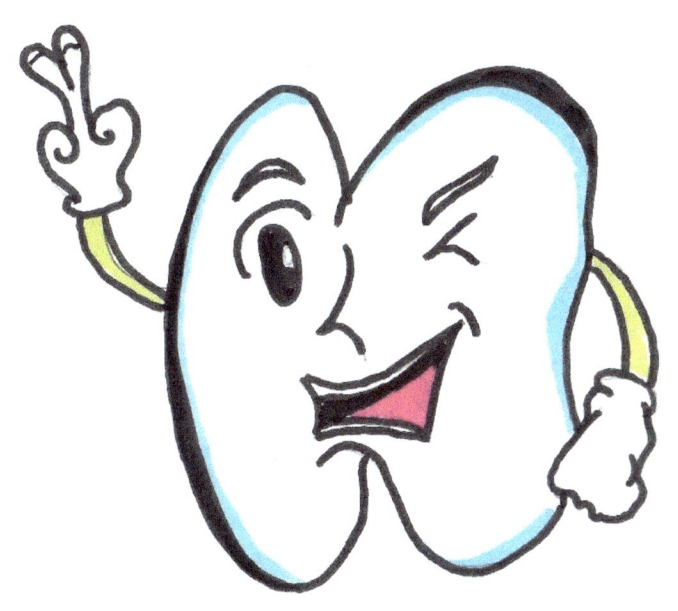

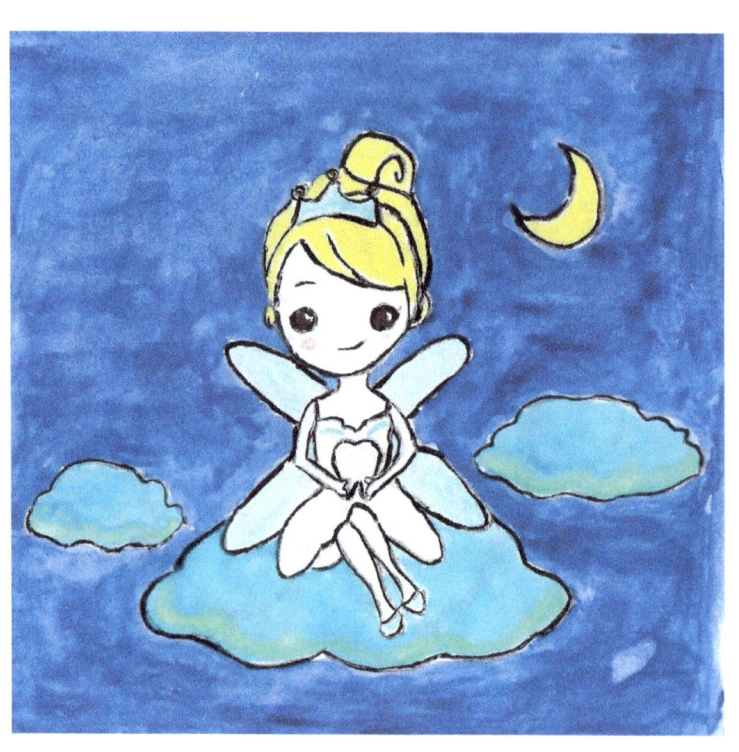

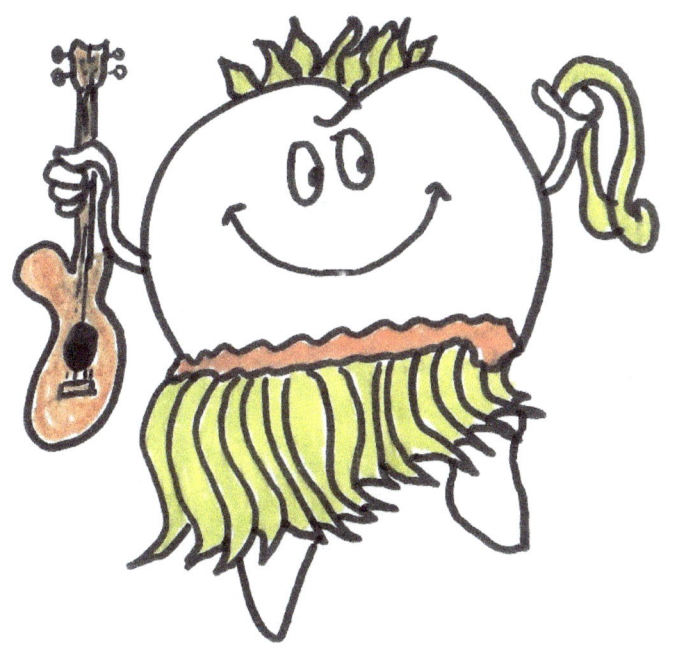

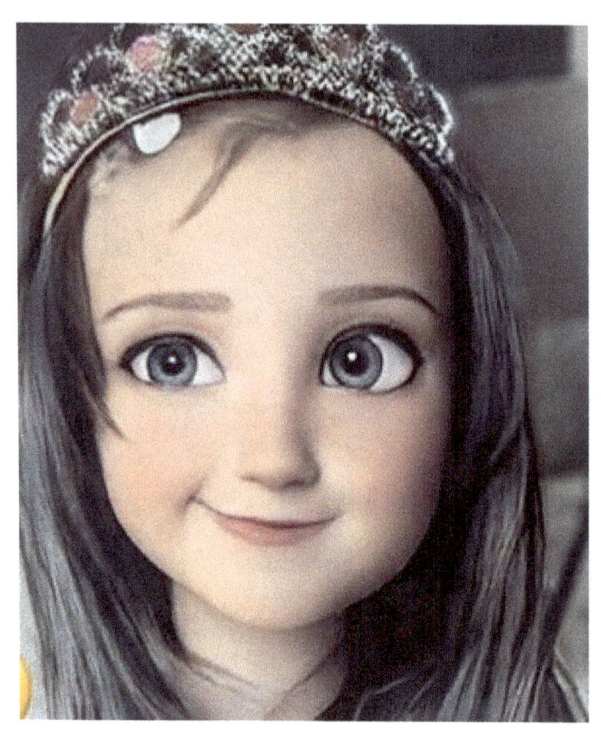

www.ingramcontent.com/pod-product-compliance
Lightning Source LLC
Chambersburg PA
CBHW071556170526

45166CB00004B/1695